THE 2023 DIABETES DIET CODE

Eat to Lose Weight and Reverse Type 2 Diabetes

Kellie J. Owsley

<u>Disclaimer</u>
The information in this book is for informational purposes only and is not intended as a substitute for professional medical advice. Always consult with a qualified healthcare professional before making any changes to your diet, lifestyle, or medication regimen.

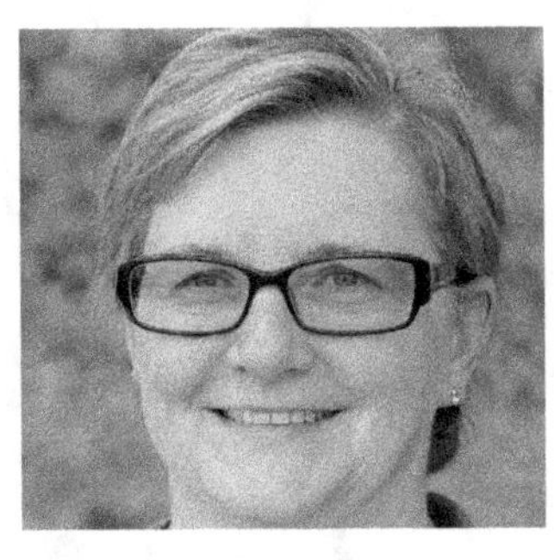

Kellie J. Owsley is a registered dietitian nutritionist (RDN) and certified diabetes care and education specialist (CDCES) who is passionate about helping people with type 2 diabetes live their healthiest lives. She has over 10 years of experience helping people manage their condition through diet and lifestyle changes, and she is the author of the book, *The 2023 Diabetes Diet Code*.

Kellie is a frequent speaker and writer on the topic of diabetes, and she is committed to providing accurate and evidence-based information to her readers. She is also a strong advocate for self-care and empowerment, and she believes that everyone with type 2 diabetes can live a long and healthy life.

Contents

Introduction

Type 2 diabetes is a chronic metabolic condition marked by hyperglycemia (excess blood sugar). Insulin resistance, or a diminished cellular response to insulin, causes it. Insulin is a hormone that controls blood sugar levels by encouraging glucose absorption into cells. Blood sugar levels increase when cells become insulin resistant, which may lead to major health consequences such as heart disease, stroke, and kidney disease.

There is no cure for type 2 diabetes, but it may be controlled by lifestyle changes such as diet and exercise, as well as medication. A balanced diet is important for people with type 2 diabetes because it helps reduce blood sugar levels and enhance insulin sensitivity.

The Diabetes Diet Code 2023 is a new dietary plan created exclusively for patients with type 2 diabetes. It is based on the most recent scientific research and has been found to help patients lose weight, reduce blood sugar levels, and reverse insulin resistance.

The 2023 Diabetes Diet Code is a high-fat, low-carbohydrate diet. It has fewer refined carbs than white bread, white rice, and pasta. It also has fewer sugary beverages and fruit juices. Avocados, nuts, and seeds are abundant in healthy fats. It also contains a lot of protein and unprocessed foods, including fruits, vegetables, and lean meats.

The 2023 Diabetes Diet Code is a versatile diet that can be customized to meet the requirements and preferences of each person. There are no hard-and-fast rules; however, it is critical to adhere to the diet's main principles.

The 2023 Diabetes Diet Code is a diet that is both safe and beneficial for those with type 2 diabetes. It may assist patients in losing weight, lowering blood sugar levels, and increasing insulin sensitivity. The diet is also adaptable and simple to follow. It is critical to consult with your doctor before embarking on the 2023

Diabetes Diet Code. They can help you decide whether the diet is suitable for you and provide support and assistance.

Chapter 1: The Science Behind the 2023 Diabetes Diet Code

Hyperglycemia (high blood sugar) is a chronic metabolic disease associated with type 2 diabetes. Insulin resistance, which is a diminished cellular response to insulin, is the root cause of it. By encouraging the absorption of glucose into cells, the hormone insulin controls blood sugar levels. Blood sugar levels increase as a result of cells losing their ability to respond to insulin, which may cause major health issues including heart disease, stroke, and kidney disease.

How does the 2023 Diabetes Diet Code work?

A low-carb, high-fat diet is part of the 2023 Diabetes Diet Code. White bread, white rice, and pasta are examples of refined carbs that are low in this food. Fruit juices and beverages with added sugar are likewise in short supply. The diet contains a lot of good fats, including those found in avocados, nuts, and seeds. It also contains a lot of protein and whole foods, including fruits, vegetables, and lean meats.

When you ingest carbs, your body converts them into glucose, the body's primary energy source. However, if you consume an excessive amount of carbs, your blood sugar levels may spike quickly. This may cause the insulin to be released, which helps to reduce blood sugar levels.

Consuming excessive amounts of carbs over time might cause insulin resistance. This occurs when your body's cells become less susceptible to the effects of insulin. As a consequence, even after eating a meal, your blood sugar levels may still be elevated.

The 2023 Diabetes Diet Code works by limiting your consumption of carbs while boosting your intake of protein and healthy fats. This raises insulin sensitivity and lowers blood sugar levels.

The Benefit of the 2023 Diabetes Diet Code

It has been shown that the 2023 Diabetes Diet Code works well in assisting those with type 2 diabetes to:

1. Reduced blood sugar levels
2. increase insulin sensitivity
3. reduce the likelihood of having renal disease, heart disease, or a stroke.
4. mood and energy levels
5. Improved sleep quality Reduced inflammatory response

The Diabetes Diet Code for 2023 is a flexible diet that may be customized to fit unique requirements and interests. Although there are no strict guidelines, it's crucial to abide by the diet's guiding principles.

- The 2023 Diabetes Diet Code's position on fat Healthy fats, like those in avocados, almonds, and seeds, may aid in increasing insulin sensitivity and reducing blood sugar levels. This is because good fats encourage satiety by slowing the blood sugar intake of carbs.

- The part that proteins play in The Diabetes Diet Secret for 2023: Building and rebuilding muscle tissue requires protein. Additionally, it supports your ability to maintain a sense of fullness and satisfaction following meals. By limiting the quantity of glucose released into the system after a meal, protein may help increase insulin sensitivity and reduce blood sugar levels.

- The 2023 Diabetes Diet Code's use of fiber: Fiber is a form of carbohydrate that the body cannot digest. It aids in reducing the rate at which glucose is absorbed into the circulation. Additionally, fiber may help reduce blood sugar levels and increase insulin sensitivity.

**Tips for adhering to the 2023 Diabetes Diet
Code:**

1. Reduce your consumption of refined carbs, such as white bread, white rice, and pasta.

2. Pick healthy fats like those in avocados, almonds, and seeds.

3. Consume lots of lean meats, poultry, fish, eggs, and beans.

4. Consume a lot of fiber-rich foods, such as fruits, vegetables, and whole grains.

5. Drink a lot of water.

It is crucial to consult your doctor before beginning the 2023 Diabetes Diet Code. They may provide you with support and direction while assisting you in determining if the diet is the best option for you.

Here are some extra pointers for adhering to the 2023 Diabetes Diet Code:

1. Plan your meals and snacks. This will assist you in avoiding harmful decisions when you are hungry.

2. More meals should be prepared at home. You will have greater control over the components in your cuisine as a result.

3. Make wholesome substitutes. For instance, choose whole-grain bread instead of white bread. Use brown rice in place of white rice.

4. Don't be hesitant to try new things. Online and in cookbooks, a wide variety of recipes and meal plans are accessible. Discover what suits your palate and needs the best.

5. Be consistent and patient. Modify your eating habits and get benefits, it takes time. If you don't notice results right away, don't lose hope. Simply keep going.

Chapter 2: The 2023 Diabetes Diet Code's Core Ideas

The diabetes diet code for 2023 calls for a high-fat, low-carbohydrate diet. It is founded on the following fundamental ideas:

- Distribution of macronutrients: The recommended macronutrient proportion for the diet is 40–50% fat, 20–30% protein, and 20–30% carbs. This indicates that you should concentrate on consuming foods high in protein, such as lean meats, poultry, fish, eggs, and legumes, as well as healthy fats, such as those included in avocados, nuts, and seeds. Various naturally occurring carbs from whole grains, vegetables, and fruits should also be a part of your diet.

- Food choices: The Diabetes Diet Code for 2023 places a strong emphasis on selecting wholesome, unadulterated meals. To do this, stay away from processed meals, sweetened beverages, and refined carbs. Eat plenty of fruits, vegetables, whole grains, lean protein, and healthy fats as opposed to refined carbohydrates.

- Meal planning: A key component of the 2023 Diabetes Diet Code is meal planning. You may use it to make healthy decisions and maintain your eating plan. Be mindful of your portion sizes when planning your meals, and make sure to incorporate a variety of foods from all the food categories.

Here are some more pointers for adhering to the 2023 Diabetes Diet Code's fundamental guidelines:

- Make a list of all the wholesome things you like to consume. When planning meals and snacks, this will assist you in making healthy decisions.

- Make more home-cooked meals. You will have greater control over the components of your diet as a result.

- Make wholesome changes. Use whole-grain bread as an example rather than white bread. Use brown rice rather than white rice.

- Analyze food labels thoroughly. Pay close attention to the serving size and the proportions of protein, fat, and carbs in each dish.

- Pay attention to your portion sizes. Even when you are consuming nutritious meals, it is easy to overeat.

- Don't be afraid to try new things. Online and in cookbooks, a wide variety of recipes and meal plans are accessible. Discover what suits both your palate and you best.

- Be persistent and patient. To alter your eating patterns and experience change, it takes time. If you don't notice results right away, don't give up. Just persevere.

You should consult your doctor before deciding whether to adopt the 2023 Diabetes Diet Code. They may provide you with support and direction while assisting you in determining if the diet is the best choice for you.

The following are some additional advantages of adhering to the main guidelines of the 2023 Diabetes Diet Code:

- An increase in insulin sensitivity Type 2 diabetes has a significant underlying root cause called insulin resistance. You may increase your insulin sensitivity and reduce your blood sugar levels by adhering to the 2023 Diabetes Diet Code's main tenets.

- Reduced inflammation: Type 2 diabetes and other chronic illnesses also have inflammation as one of their underlying causes. You may lessen inflammation and enhance your general health by consuming a balanced diet full of anti-inflammatory nutrients.

- Weight loss: If you are obese or overweight, lowering your weight may help you better regulate your blood sugar levels and lower your chance of developing further type 2 diabetes issues. A healthy weight may be attained and maintained with the aid of the 2023 Diabetes Diet Code.

If you're seeking a nutritious diet that will help you control your type 2 diabetes, consider the 2023 Diabetes Diet Code as a fantastic choice. To find out whether this diet is good for you, speak with your doctor right away.

Chapter 3: The 2023 Diabetes Diet Code and Intermittent Fasting

A common eating behavior called intermittent fasting includes frequent, brief fasts. It is more of a system for planning your meals and snacks than it is a particular diet. Although there are many different ways to practice intermittent fasting, most of them entail going without food for some time each day or eating just once every few days.

Numerous health advantages of intermittent fasting have been shown, including better blood sugar regulation, less inflammation, and weight reduction. It is a common option for those with type 2 diabetes because of these advantages.

How does a periodic fasting process work?

Your body enters a condition called ketosis when you fast. When your body is in ketosis, it switches to using fat for energy instead of carbs. This is because when you don't eat, your blood sugar levels fall. Your body responds by releasing hormones that tell your liver to start converting stored fat into ketones.

For the body, ketones are a healthy and effective source of energy. Additionally, they have been linked to a range of health advantages, including increased insulin sensitivity, decreased inflammation, and weight reduction.

Intermittent fasting's benefits for patients with type 2 diabetes

People with type 2 diabetes have been proven to benefit from intermittent fasting in a variety of ways, including:

- Increased insulin sensitivity and better blood sugar regulation are two benefits of intermittent fasting. This is because intermittent fasting encourages the synthesis of ketones and reduces inflammation.

- reduced inflammation One of the main underlying causes of type 2 diabetes and other chronic illnesses is inflammation. It has been shown that intermittent fasting lowers inflammation everywhere throughout the body.

- Weight loss: If you are obese or overweight, lowering your weight may help you better regulate your blood sugar levels and lower your chance of developing further type 2 diabetes issues. By consuming fewer calories and encouraging the combustion of fat stores, intermittent fasting may aid in weight loss.

- increased cardiovascular fitness It has been shown that intermittent fasting improves cardiovascular health by reducing blood pressure and cholesterol levels.

- Reduced risk of Alzheimer's disease: It has been shown that intermittent fasting protects the brain from harm and lowers the chance of getting Alzheimer's.

Various forms of sporadic fasting

Intermittent fasting may be done in a variety of ways. Among the most well-liked techniques are:

- The 16/8 technique: This approach calls for an eight-hour window of eating followed by a 16-hour daily fast.

- The 5:2 approach: In this approach, you eat normally for 5 days out of every 7 and limit your caloric intake to 500–600 calories on the other 2 days.

- The eat-stop-eat strategy: This strategy entails a 24-hour fast once or twice every week.

Start-up instructions for intermittent fasting

Starting cautiously with intermittent fasting is crucial if you are new to it. It's also crucial to pay attention to your body's signals and break your fast if you feel sick.

Here are some pointers for beginning an intermittent fast:

- Start by going 12 hours without eating. As you become more acclimated to fasting, you may lengthen it progressively.
- Eat solely within a certain time of every day. You may eat, for instance, between 12:00 and 8:00 p.m.

- During your dining window, stay away from processed meals, sweet beverages, and harmful fats.

- During your fasting intervals, be sure to drink enough water. Black coffee, unsweetened tea, and water are all sensible choices.

Before beginning intermittent fasting, be careful to discuss any underlying medical issues with your doctor. They may aid in your assessment of the safety of this eating regimen for you.
The Diabetes Diet Code of 2023 and intermittent fasting

The Diabetes Diet Code for 2023 might include intermittent fasting. You may, for instance, adhere to a 16/8 fasting schedule, eating only during an 8-hour window each day. You would concentrate on eating wholesome meals like unprocessed carbs, lean protein, and healthy fats within your eating window.

The 2023 Diabetes Diet Code's advantages—such as increased blood sugar management, less inflammation, and weight loss—can be enhanced with intermittent fasting. The outcomes of continuing research on intermittent fasting and type 2 diabetes are encouraging. In a recent study, researchers discovered that for type 2 diabetics looking to improve blood sugar control and lose weight, intermittent fasting was equally as successful as a calorie-restricted diet.

Chapter Four: Managing the 2023 Diabetes Diet Code with Other Medications

You could be taking medication to control your blood sugar levels if you have type 2 diabetes. The best way to combine the 2023 Diabetes Diet Code with your other medications is to discuss this with your doctor.

When using the 2023 diabetic diet code while taking diabetic medications, there are a few factors to keep in mind:

- Know the negative consequences of your prescription drugs. The 2023 Diabetes Diet Code might be challenging to adhere to if some drugs induce weight gain or other negative effects. For instance, sulfonylureas might result in hypoglycemia (low blood sugar), while insulin can lead to weight gain.

- Adjust your medication dosages with your doctor as necessary. Your doctor may be able to change your prescription or reduce the dose if you are having problems adhering to the 2023 Diabetes Diet Code due to your medicines.

- Regularly check your blood sugar levels. To ensure that your blood sugar levels are under control and that you are not suffering any difficulties, it is crucial to frequently test your blood sugar levels.

- Be persistent and patient. Finding the ideal balance between the 2023 Diabetes Diet Code and your medications may take some time. If you don't notice results right away, don't give up. Just persevere.

The following advice is particular to using the 2023 diabetic diet code in conjunction with popular diabetic medications:

- **Insulin:** A hormone called insulin aids in the process of your cells absorbing glucose from the blood. Depending on your diet, you may need to change the dose of insulin you're taking. For instance, you may need to lower your insulin dose if you are consuming fewer carbs. When using the 2023 Diabetes Diet Code, make sure to discuss how to modify your insulin dose with your doctor.

- **Sulfonylureas:** A group of drugs called sulfonylureas stimulates the pancreas to produce more insulin as its mode of action. When following the 2023 Diabetes Diet Code, you may need to lower your sulfonylurea dose or switch to a different kind of medicine. This is due to the possibility of hypoglycemia while using sulfonylureas in conjunction with a low-carbohydrate diet.

- **Metformin:** Metformin is a drug that aids in lowering the quantity of glucose the liver produces. When adhering to the 2023 Diabetes Diet Code, metformin use is usually considered safe. However, it's crucial to be aware of metformin's possible adverse effects, which include nausea and diarrhea.

- **GLP-1 receptor agonists:** GLP-1 receptor agonists are a family of drugs that imitate the actions of GLP-1, a hormone that naturally lowers blood sugar and encourages satiety. In general, it's okay to use GLP-1 receptor agonists while adhering to the 2023 Diabetes Diet Code. They may, however, result in negative side effects such as nausea, vomiting, and diarrhea.

- **SGLT2 inhibitors:** A family of drugs known as SGLT2 inhibitors stimulates the kidneys to eliminate more glucose in the urine. In general, using SGLT2 inhibitors while following the 2023 Diabetes Diet Code is safe. They could, however, result in negative side effects, including dehydration and urinary tract infections.

It's crucial to maintain a healthy lifestyle in addition to adhering to the 2023 diabetic diet code and taking your diabetic medications as directed. This involves controlling stress, taking regular exercise, and getting adequate sleep. You can control your type 2 diabetes and enhance your general health by using these suggestions.

Additional advice for using the 2023 Diabetes Diet Code with different drugs is provided below:

- Keep a food and glucose journal. You may monitor your blood sugar levels and look for trends in them. Additionally, you may utilize this journal to update your doctor on your progress.

- Learn all you can about the 2023 Diabetes Diet Code and diabetes. Both online and in libraries, there are a ton of materials accessible. The more prepared you are to manage your condition, the more you will know about diabetes and the diet.

- Sign up for a support group. You may get emotional support and useful information from other individuals living with diabetes in support groups.

You may improve your general health and manage the 2023 Diabetes Diet Code with your other medicines by paying attention to these suggestions.

Chapter Five: Common Challenges and How to Overcome Them

It might be difficult to follow the 2023 Diabetes Diet Code at times. People who follow the diet often encounter a variety of difficulties, such as:

- Hunger and cravings: When eating a low-carbohydrate diet, it might be challenging to withstand the desire for sweets and carbs. However, there are a variety of strategies for controlling hunger and cravings, including eating regular meals and snacks, getting adequate sleep, and drinking a lot of water.

- Finding healthy meal alternatives while eating out might be challenging. However, there are some things you can do to make healthy choices, such as finding restaurants that provide healthy selections, inquiring about the ingredients in meals, and bringing your food.

- Motivation: Maintaining motivation to follow a diet, particularly over an extended period, may be challenging. Setting attainable objectives, finding a support network, and rewarding yourself for your accomplishments are a few strategies you may use to maintain your motivation.

Here are some concrete suggestions for overcoming typical difficulties while using the 2023 Diabetes Diet Code:

1. Hunger and cravings

- Eat often throughout the day to maintain steady blood sugar levels and avoid cravings.
- To keep hydrated and satisfied, drink plenty of water.
- Get enough rest. You're less likely to feel cravings and hunger when you're well-rested.

- Avoid processed meals, fizzy drinks, and refined carbs. These meals may increase cravings and make it challenging to maintain a diet.
- Discover some tasty, healthy snacks. It will be simpler to control the desire for unhealthy meals as a result.
- If a need does strike, attempt to divert your attention by doing something else, such as taking a stroll, listening to music, or chatting with a friend.

2. Dine outside

- To learn more about the ingredients in the meals, call ahead of time.
- Look for eateries that provide grilled chicken or fish, salads, and steamed veggies as healthy alternatives.
- If there isn't a meal without sauce or dressing on the menu, request it instead.
- If you're going to a restaurant that doesn't offer many healthy selections, bring your food.

3. Staying motivated

- Set attainable objectives. Avoid attempting too much change too fast. Start by implementing little adjustments, such as increasing daily vegetable consumption by one serving or avoiding sugary beverages.
- Find a network of support. Ask for their support by discussing your objectives with your friends, family, and/or doctor.
- Gratify yourself for your development. Reward yourself with something you like when you accomplish a goal.

It might be difficult to follow the 2023 Diabetes Diet Code, but it is feasible to do so and reach your objectives. The advice given above will help you position yourself for success.

Here are a few more suggestions for overcoming typical difficulties while using the 2023 Diabetes Diet Code:

- Never hesitate to seek assistance. Speak with your doctor or a certified dietitian if you're finding it difficult to stick to the diet. They might provide you with assistance and direction.

- Never give up. Everyone errs sometimes. Don't berate yourself if you make a mistake. Simply get back up and try again.

- Keep in mind why you are doing this. Are you following the 2023 Diabetes Diet Code to lower your risk of problems, enhance your blood sugar management, or for any other reason? You'll remain motivated if you keep your objectives in mind.

Chapter Six: Exercise and the 2023 Diabetes Diet Code

A crucial component of controlling type 2 diabetes is exercise. It helps to decrease the risk of complications, raise insulin sensitivity, and lower blood sugar levels. Exercise may aid in weight reduction, which can enhance blood sugar management and lower the likelihood of problems.

People with type 2 diabetes are advised by the 2023 Diabetes Diet Code to engage in at least 150 minutes of moderate-intensity aerobic activity or 75 minutes of vigorous-intensity aerobic activity per week. Additionally, two times a week, strength-training activities are recommended for those with type 2 diabetes.

Exercises that fall under the category of moderate-intensity aerobics include brisk walking, bicycling, swimming, and dancing. Running, jogging, and participating in sports are examples of vigorous-intensity aerobic exercise.

Workouts for building strength include utilizing resistance bands, lifting weights, and bodyweight workouts.

It's crucial to begin cautiously while exercising if you've never done it before, then gradually build up your exercises' length and intensity over time. Before beginning any new workout regimen, it's also advisable to speak with your doctor, particularly if you have any underlying medical issues.

The following advice will help you include exercise in your daily routine while adhering to the 2023 Diabetes Diet Code:

- Find things you like to do. A negative attitude makes it less likely that you will continue with an activity.

- Set attainable objectives. Try not to do too much too quickly. Start with simple objectives, like going for three 30-minute walks each week.

- Include exercise in your daily regimen. Just like any other essential appointment, plan time in your day for exercise.

- Get a workout partner. Having a workout partner helps keep you accountable and motivated.

- Be aware of your body. Don't exert too much effort. If you have pain, stop and take a break.

The 2023 Diabetes Diet Code and controlling type 2 diabetes both heavily emphasize exercise. The aforementioned advice will help you incorporate exercise into your daily routine and enhance your general health and well-being.

Additional advantages of exercise for those with type 2 diabetes include the following:

- Blood pressure, cholesterol, and blood sugar are all reduced with exercise, which also lowers the risk of heart disease and stroke. Heart disease and stroke, two of the main causes of mortality in patients with type 2 diabetes, may be lowered as a result of this.

- Increased energy and mood: Endorphins, which improve mood, are released during exercise. Exercise may also aid in bettering sleep, which can result in more energy throughout the day.

- Reduced risk of depression: Type 2 diabetics are more likely to experience depression. Exercise has been shown to help ease depression symptoms and elevate moods in general.

Before beginning any new fitness program, if you are new to exercising, it is crucial to speak with your doctor. They can assist you in choosing the best workout style and level for you.

Chapter Seven: Living with Type 2 Diabetes: Coping and Support

Living with type 2 diabetes may sometimes be difficult. Maintaining control over your blood sugar levels, eating well, and exercising regularly might be challenging. You could also struggle with emotional issues, including stress, anxiety, and despair.

Managing the difficulties of type 2 diabetes
Here are some suggestions for overcoming the difficulties caused by type 2 diabetes:

- Do some research on type 2 diabetes. Your ability to handle your disease will improve the more you are aware of it. Both online and in libraries, there are a ton of materials accessible.

- Find a network of support. Tell your doctor, family, and friends about your struggles. Additionally, you may become a member of a type 2 diabetes support group. You may get emotional support and useful information from other individuals who are dealing with the same problem in support groups.

- Create effective coping strategies. Look for appropriate coping mechanisms for stress and anxiety. This can include getting some exercise, unwinding, or spending time with close friends and family.

- Never hesitate to seek assistance. Speak to your doctor or a mental health professional if you're having trouble managing the difficulties of having type 2 diabetes. They might provide you with assistance and direction.

Here are some more pointers for managing type 2 diabetes while leading a healthy life:

- Ensure your well-being. Be sure to obtain adequate rest, maintain a nutritious diet, and engage in regular exercise.

- Regularly check your blood sugar levels. This will enable you to see any trends and alter your food and exercise routine as necessary.

- Be equipped to handle crises. Always carry insulin and a glucose meter in case your blood sugar levels go too low.

- Never be reluctant to discuss any concerns you may have with your doctor. They are available to support you as you live a healthy life and manage your diabetes.

Here are some more suggestions for managing type 2 diabetes:

- Set attainable objectives. Avoid attempting too much change too fast. Start by implementing little adjustments, such as increasing daily vegetable consumption by one serving or avoiding sugary beverages.

- Find some tasty, healthy snacks. It will be simpler to control the desire for unhealthy meals as a result.

- Gratify yourself for your development. Reward yourself with something you like when you accomplish a goal.

- Never give up. Everyone errs sometimes. Don't berate yourself if you make a mistake. Simply get back up and try again.

- Keep in mind why you are doing this. Do you lead a healthy lifestyle for weight loss, better blood sugar regulation, less risk of problems, or another reason? You'll remain motivated if you keep your objectives in mind.

Despite the difficulties of having type 2 diabetes, it is still possible to live a long and healthy life. You can control your diabetes and enhance your general well-being by using the preceding advice.

Conclusion

Type 2 diabetes is a chronic metabolic condition that may have serious health consequences. You can control your type 2 diabetes and live a long and healthy life by following the 2023 Diabetes Diet Code and implementing other lifestyle adjustments.

The 2023 Diabetes Diet Code's main points are as follows:

- Consume healthy fats like those found in avocados, almonds, and seeds.

- Protein-rich foods include lean meats, poultry, fish, eggs, and lentils.

- Consume a variety of unprocessed carbs, such as fruits, vegetables, and whole grains, throughout your diet.

- Refined carbs, fizzy drinks, and processed meals should all be avoided.

- Regularly monitor your blood sugar levels and make necessary changes to your diet and exercise routine.

The 2023 Diabetes Diet Code has the following additional advantages:

- **Reduced risk** of cardiovascular disease and stroke

- Improvements in mood and energy levels

- Depression risk is reduced.

- Loss of weight (if desired)

Tips for living with type 2 diabetes include:

- Learn about type 2 diabetes and the Diabetes Diet Code 2023.

- Find a support system for type 2 diabetes friends, family members, or other individuals.

- Create appropriate stress and anxiety coping techniques.

- Don't be hesitant to seek your doctor or a mental health professional for assistance.

- Take care of yourself by obtaining adequate rest, eating nutritious food, and exercising regularly.

- Always have a glucose meter and insulin on hand in case of an emergency.

- Don't be scared to discuss any concerns you have with your doctor.

Keep in mind that you are not alone. Millions of individuals suffer from type 2 diabetes. There are also several resources available to assist you in managing your disease and living a healthy lifestyle. Consult your doctor for the best resources for you.

Here are some more views on how to live with type 2 diabetes:

It is critical to have a good mindset and concentrate on what you can manage. This covers your eating habits, exercise routine, and stress levels. You may lower your risk of issues and live a long and full life by making good choices.

It's also important to be patient and realistic. It takes time to become used to a new way of life and to notice benefits. Don't be disheartened if you don't notice instant benefits. Simply persevere and be patient.

Finally, congratulate yourself on your accomplishments. Even little accomplishments, such as eating a nutritious meal or going for a stroll, are worthy of celebration. You will remain motivated and on track if you recognize your achievements.

Although living with type 2 diabetes might be difficult, it is possible to live a long and healthy life. You can control your diabetes and enhance your general well-being by following the guidelines above.